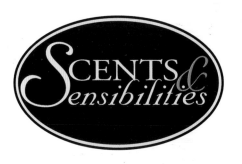

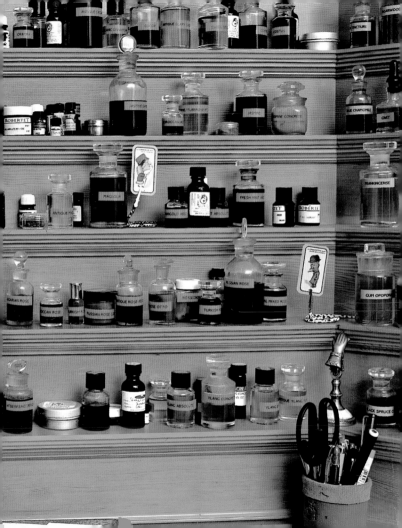

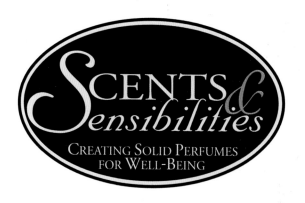

SCENTS & Sensibilities

CREATING SOLID PERFUMES
FOR WELL-BEING

MANDY AFTEL

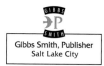

Gibbs Smith, Publisher
Salt Lake City

All illustrations, memorabilia, cases, and compacts
courtesy of the Mandy Aftel collection.

First Edition
09 08 07 06 05   5 4 3 2 1

Published by
Gibbs Smith, Publisher
P.O. Box 667
Layton, Utah 84041

Orders: 1.800.748.5439
www.gibbs-smith.com

Designed by Dawn DeVries Sokol
Printed and bound in Hong Kong

Library of Congress Cataloging-in-Publication Data

Aftel, Mandy.
Scents & sensibilities : creating solid perfumes for well-being / Mandy
Aftel.— 1st ed.
p. cm.
ISBN 1-58685-738-X
1. Perfumes. I. Title: Scents and sensibilities. II. Title.
TP983.A725 2005
668'.54—dc22
                              2004023376

For Patty Curtan

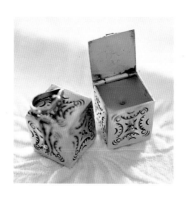

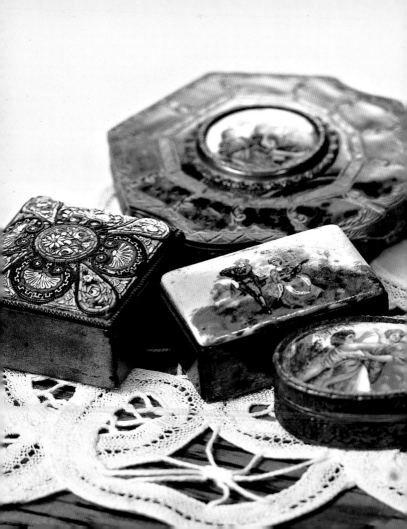

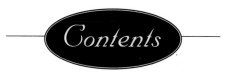

Contents

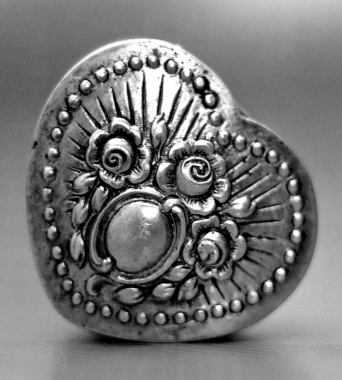

ACKNOWLEDGMENTS

I would like to thank a few people for their help and support: the people at Gibbs Smith, Publisher—Jennifer Grillone, Alison Einerson, Laura Ayrey, Suzanne Taylor, and Gibbs Smith—for making the whole experience of writing and publishing this book a pleasure; my agent, Amy Williams, for her belief in my work; Randi Nagahori, my assistant, for her hard work and great spirit; Jody Hanson for making my perfumes look so beautiful and for her friendship; Susan Griffin, Elissa Schappell, William T. Vollman, and Andy Eales, for their love, support, and kindness; Becky Saletan for being the best friend I have ever had; and my appreciation and love to my daughter, Chloe, always and forever.

$\mathcal{I}$NTRODUCTION

SCENTS ARE LINKED TO EMOTION, and perfume has been known to have a powerful effect on our sensibilities. People have used solid perfumes to soothe the psyche, entice a lover, transform an intimate environment, enliven the spirit, and recall a precious memory. Solid perfume has a long history of bringing well-being, comfort, protection, allure, and pleasure. Much like an early form of aromatherapy, solid perfumes have been used for treatment as well as pleasure throughout history.

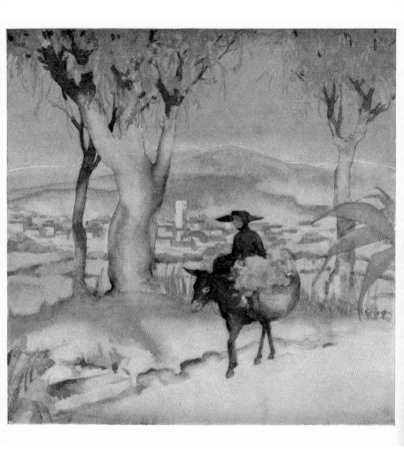

Transporting harvested flowers in Grasse, France.

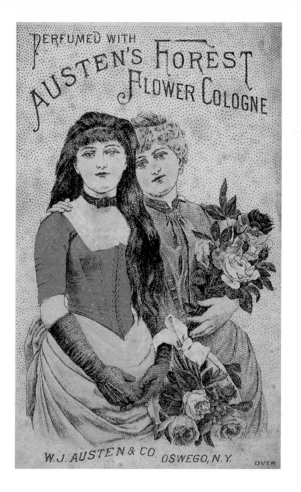

To make solid perfume, oil-based perfume is combined with melted wax and then poured into a container where it solidifies. Solid perfume is portable and can be transported easily, even secretly carried on the body in a pendant, charm, or ring. One of the ingenious aspects of solid perfumes is that

The experience of applying solid perfume creates positive emotions.

you can keep it close at hand and take it with you without worrying about it spilling. Unobtrusive to apply, it is easy to carry in a handbag, briefcase, or backpack.

In addition to its aroma, the experience of applying solid perfume creates positive emotions; earthy and sensual, its application creates a sensation completely different from spraying a cologne or dabbing a liquid perfume. Solid perfume will scent only you, not the environment around you. The perfume is often housed in small and beautiful containers that grow more precious and treasured with use.

Because of its portability, solid perfume is easily incorporated into your life, soothing you in situations where you feel stressed or anxious. Smoothing it on your skin immediately brings you pleasure and a sense of well-being that is both comforting and pampering. Applying solid perfume can become a discreet, quiet, pleasurable ritual in your life—the sensuality of rubbing your fingers across its salve-like texture, the pleasure of smelling and then applying the fragrance. The feeling in the hand of the beautiful container increases your sense of individuality and pleasure. When you have used up the perfume,

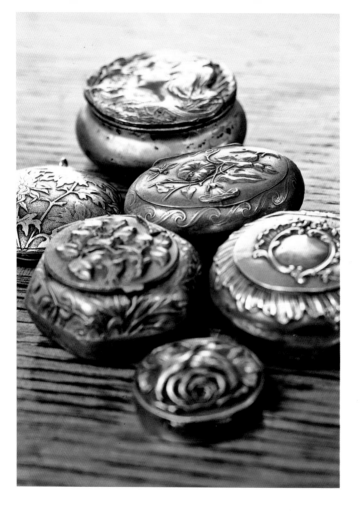

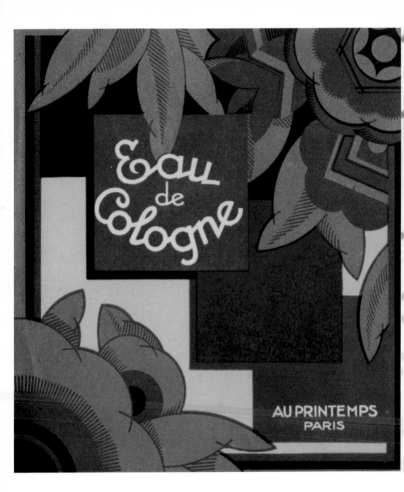

instead of throwing away the container, as is done with most cosmetics, you can simply refill it with a new perfume. Then your attachment is not only to the perfume but to the case as well.

When I am in a situation that I find stressful, such as bumper-to-bumper traffic or dealing with

---

Applying solid perfume can become a discreet, quiet, pleasurable ritual in your life.

---

people that are difficult, I often, even without thinking about it, reach into my bag and take out my solid perfume to rub a bit across the back of my hands. Studies have shown that 80 percent of American women report that they are stressed out and that relaxation at work and at home would improve their daily life. Using solid perfumes is a simple activity to incorporate into your life for reducing stress. When you're in a situation that makes you nervous or frustrated, you can reconnect with yourself and find pleasure in simply applying perfume and inhaling deeply. Over time, just a whiff of your special fragrance can help you to become calmer and more grounded.

Fragrances can be used to change your mood. Some perfumes elevate your mood, others calm anxious and frenetic nerves, and still others create a feeling of joy and well-being. In this book, you will learn how to make your own solid perfumes. You will find recipes for increasing your sense of tranquility, joy, sensuality, and refreshment, as well as learn how to create perfumes that are the perfect blend of essences for you.

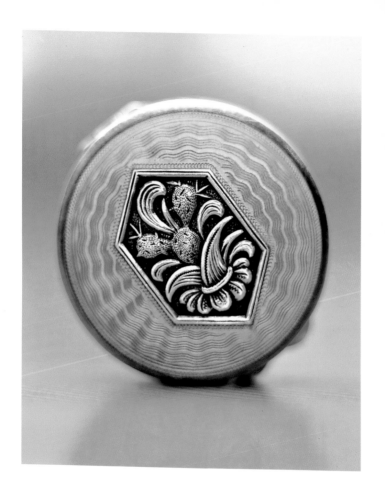

A BRIEF HISTORY OF SOLID PERFUME

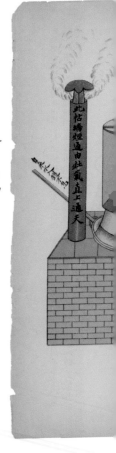

THROUGHOUT TIME DIFFERENT CULTURES have used perfumes to enhance their lives and sense of well-being. Solid perfumes have a long and varied history and were some of the earliest perfumes known to man.

Ancient Egypt

The earliest perfumes were called *unguents*, which referred both to

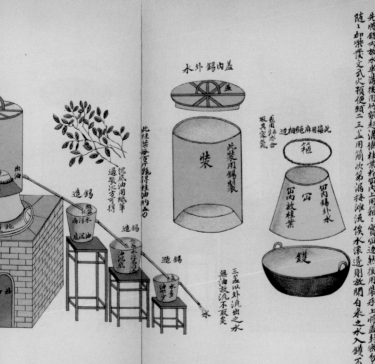

Chinese Still for Cassia Oil.

蓋內錫外水

盒

此裝用錫製

裝

此相範席用攝此

義用歸茱
取其窖氣

邊相範席用攝此

插

窖內錫外
窖內放桂葉

鑊

此桂葉每蒸餾得油約五斤

泥底油用紙筆
過數淨方可得

造錫

熱汕
兩浮水
底沉油

造錫

流底

造錫

水多
油少
浮少

三盆以外流出之水
無油放流不取矣

水

出油

先將鑵內放水半滿後用竹架起滿鑵桂業於鑵內用箱二實卽邊裝
隨、如裝葉文武火預頂二三盆用箱次第滿接瀉流候水滾透則放開自來之水入鑵不歇水
然後用柴承上將蓋封寔勿令洩氣

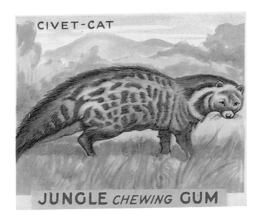

CIVET-CAT

JUNGLE *CHEWING* GUM

oil-based perfume and semisolid perfumed ointment. Thirty-five hundred years ago in Egypt, women wore solid perfumes on their heads in the form of a cone, called an unguent or scent cone. A surviving picture of an ancient banquet depicts guests and servants with unguent cones on their heads, as well as servants ministering to the guests with a bowl of solid unguent, a handful of which would be placed on a

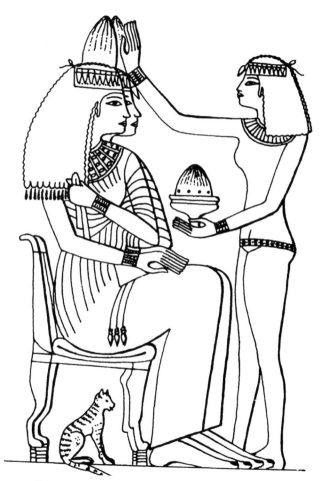

Egyptians with unguent cones.

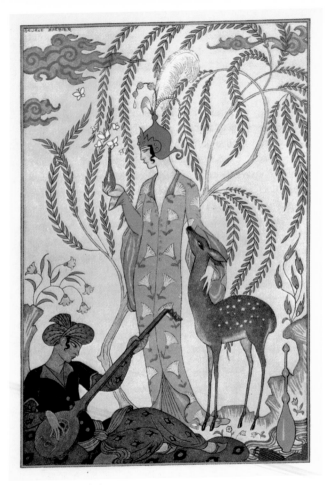

Woman with musk deer.

guest's head.* To make unguents, plant parts and flowers were steeped in fat, which was then shaped into cones. Sometimes the cone was made of tallow impregnated with myrrh. The cone was placed on the head so that as the heat of the day melted the fat, it would trickle down over the head and body, covering the wearer with fragrance. In tomb paintings, these cones are similar to halos in early Christian art, signifying the state of blessedness.

Ancient Rome

In the baths of ancient Rome—which functioned like today's spa—was an area called the unguentarium. In the unguentarium, thick, ointment-like perfumes were smeared liberally on the body. Generally, they consisted of one specific scent in an animal-fat base, (usually

*Lisa Manniche, *Sacred Luxuries: Fragrance, Aromatherapy, and Cosmetics in Ancient Egypt* (Ithaca, New York: Cornell University Press, 1999), 94–96.

hog's lard).* The wealthy often brought custom scents made exclusively for them. At the beginning of the process, the bather's body was freely anointed with cheap, strong, fragrant oils; at the end of the process,

---

The wealthy often brought custom scents made exclusively for them.

---

slaves carrying little vases of alabaster, bronze, or terra-cotta full of perfumed oils rubbed the oils over every part of the bather's body—on the hair, the breast, the legs, and sometimes even the soles of the feet.

Pomanders

The first widespread form of aromatic jewelry was the pomander, which consisted of an elaborate

*Ivan Day, *Perfumery with Herbs* (London: Darton, Longman, and Todd Limited, 1979), 10.

filigreed gold or silver ball worn on a chain around the neck or wrist. Some pomanders were sectioned like apple slices, with a different perfume in each section. The ball was filled with solid perfume, often containing ambergris—the legendary perfume ingredient derived from whales—giving rise to the term *pomme amber* or amber apple.

To prepare the pomander mixture, the resins—usually benzoin and labdanum—would be melted in a pan and then the ambergris would be added. While the mixture was still pliable, it was rolled into a ball in the palms of the hands or pressed into pomander molds. In other recipes, rose, spikenard, and myrrh were all pounded together in a ball and then dried in the shade. The ambergris was used to "fix" the mixture, or make the scent of the other ingredients last longer.

Smelling Boxes

From the Middle Ages to the Renaissance, precious aromatics, like ambergris, were placed inside small boxes carried by both men and women and sniffed to ward off the unwholesome smell of the streets and rooms. Sometimes the smelling boxes were pomanders with separate compartments, so the aromas could be enjoyed singly or in combination. These silver or gold boxes came in various shapes, such as books, hearts, dogs, fish, or snails. One interesting smelling box was the knob at the top of a doctor's walking stick, which was filled with aromatic substances and used when visiting plague victims or patients in infectious situations.*

---

*Edmund Launert, *Perfume and Pomanders* (Munich: Georg D. W. Callwey, 1987), 25.

Perfumed Rings, Brooches, Pendants, and Charms

The possibilities for solid perfume in jewelry are end-less, and their history is well documented in Annette Green and Linda Dyett's sumptuous book, *The Secrets of Aromatic Jewelry.** Brooches and pendants with cavities filled with solid perfume were lovely worn close to the heart. A ring could contain a hinged bezel, beneath which was a special compartment where aromatics (such as leaves, spices, or musk) could be stored. As the ancients used perfumes in brooches, rings, pendants, and charms, so can we incorporate the same pleasurable effects of solid perfume in jewelry today.

*Paris: Flammarion, 1998.

NATURAL ESSENCES

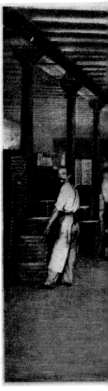

NATURAL ESSENCES ARE LIKE THE
ATOMS of creating a fragrance, the
building blocks with which complex and
evocative scents are made. The odors of
plants reside in different parts of the
plant: sometimes in the rind of the fruit,
as with blood orange and pink grapefruit;
sometimes in the roots, as with iris and
the grass known as vetiver; sometimes in
the woody stem, as with cedarwood or
sandalwood. Sometimes they reside in the

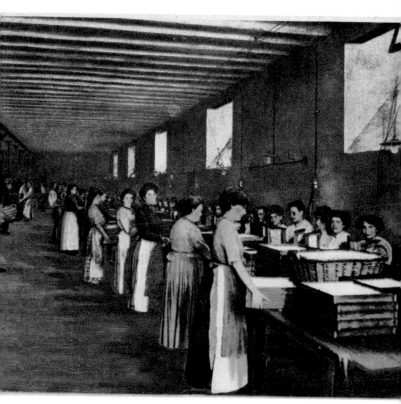

Scent-harvesting jasmine.

bark, as with cinnamon; sometimes in the leaves, as with mint, patchouli, and thyme; sometimes in the seeds, as with tonka bean and ambrette; and sometimes in the flower, as with rose and jasmine.

Essential Oils

Essential oils are the largest category of fragrance materials, and the most widely available, thanks to the tremendous popularity of aromatherapy. Most of the oils come from a process called distillation, except for the oils extracted from citrus fruits, which are rendered by simple pressing. Steam distillation is the more common and gentle method for the extraction of essential oils. Small pieces of oil-bearing plant material are placed in the still. Steam is passed though the still, causing the oil to vaporize. The mixture of steam and oil vapor then passes through a condenser and returns to a liquid phase, where the oil and water separate. The oil rendered is the essential oil.

Concretes and Absolutes

Many natural flower oils are rendered from fresh flowers by solvent extraction. Because the flowers give off a great deal of waxy material, the process yields a so-called concrete, which is semisolid. Concretes have great staying power but softness to their aroma. They are perfect for making solid perfume.

In solvent extraction, flowers are placed on racks in a hermetically sealed container. A liquid solvent, usually hexane, is circulated over the flowers to dissolve the essential oils. This produces a solid waxy paste, the concrete. The concrete is then repeatedly treated with pure alcohol (ethanol), which dissolves the wax and yields the intensely aromatic liquid known as an absolute. Absolutes are floral essences at their truest and most concentrated. They are much more lasting than essential oils and have an intensity and fineness to their aroma that is unequalled. They are the most expensive perfumery ingredients.

Resins and Balsams

Resins are the viscous, solid, or semisolid gums derived from trees, such as frankincense and myrrh, or dry lichens growing on the bark of oaks and other trees, such as oakmoss. They are of great use to the perfumer for their staying power.

Balsams are raw, resinous, semisolid, or viscous materials exuded by trees, usually through incisions in the bark. They often have a cinnamon or vanilla scent. They are almost completely soluble in alcohol, and, like resins, they help to "fix" a perfume and make it last.

A NOTE ABOUT SAFETY

Some natural essences have been known to cause allergic reactions when applied directly to the skin. Others have provoked adverse reactions when used in very large quantities, ingested orally, or rubbed into the skin. Even though natural essences in solid perfume are diluted in jojoba oil and beeswax, if you are prone to allergies or have sensitive skin, it may be advisable to try a patch test to see if a given oil is problematic for you. Apply one drop of the oil in question to the inside of your forearm and cover it with an adhesive strip. After a few hours, check for redness or irritation.

It is best to avoid natural essences on the skin during pregnancy. They can pass from the skin into the bloodstream, and some of them may cross the placental barrier. The International Fragrance Association (IFRA) has compiled a list of recommended guidelines for commercial perfumers that is updated periodically. You can find it on the web at www.ifraorg.org/guidelines.asp.

Top, Middle, and Base Notes

Perfume essences (I use the term *essences* to cover essential oils, absolutes, concretes, resins, and balsams) are classified into top, middle, and base notes according to their relative volatility, or the speed with which they diffuse into the air. Or we could look at this quality from the opposite perspective and say that they are grouped according to their relative tenacity, which refers to the length of time they remain fragrant on the skin before they fade away entirely. The residual odor left after the more volatile components of an essence have evaporated is the dryout note.

Top notes, or head notes, reach our sense of smell first, forming the scent's initial impression and then quickly dissipating. They are ease to use, inexpensive,

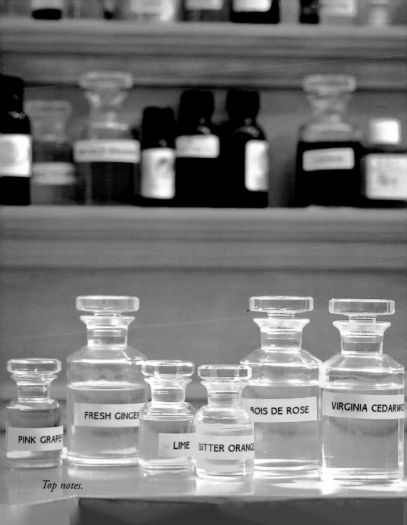

Top notes.

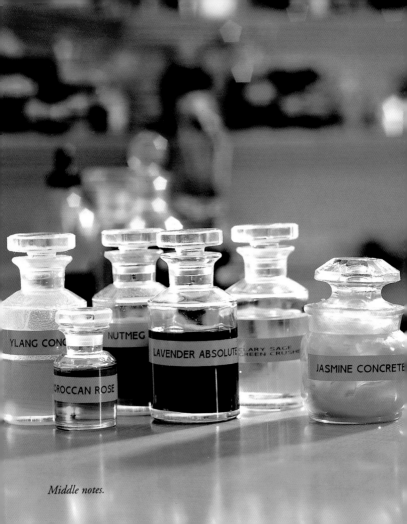

YLANG CONC NUTMEG

OROCCAN ROSE

LAVENDER ABSOLUTE CLARY SAGE GREEN CRUSHE

JASMINE CONCRETE

Middle notes.

uncomplicated, and spontaneous. Many of them are familiar from cooking: herbs and spices such as coriander, spearmint, black pepper, cardamom, juniper, basil, tarragon; and citruses such as lime, bitter orange, blood orange, tangerine, pink grapefruit. The role of a top note is to lend definition and give perfume a starting point.

Flowers, such as geranium, rose, jasmine, orange flower, tuberose, violet leaf, and ylang ylang, have always provided the most precious middle notes, or heart notes. Heady, dramatic, intense, sometimes sickly sweet, heart notes give body to blends, imparting warmth and fullness, and they bring out the best in the other notes.

Intense and profound, base notes evolve over the course of hours or even days. They are often thick and syrupy, and most are derived from bark (sandalwood), roots (angelica), resins (labdanum), lichens (oakmoss), saps (benzoin, Peru balsam), and grasses (vetiver).

Because the base note is the scent that lasts the longest on the skin, it mixes most deeply with the wearer's body chemistry. Individual body chemistries react differently with the same perfume elements. Some bring out the florals, some the spices. The skin is a base under the base, and thus base notes form the most intimate connection between perfume and wearer. They articulate the perfume's lasting character, its final perceptible note after the others have evaporated.

Essential oils are frequently top notes, whereas absolutes and concretes are middle and base notes. Many plants, including lavender and clary sage, can yield their fragrance in all three forms, each form

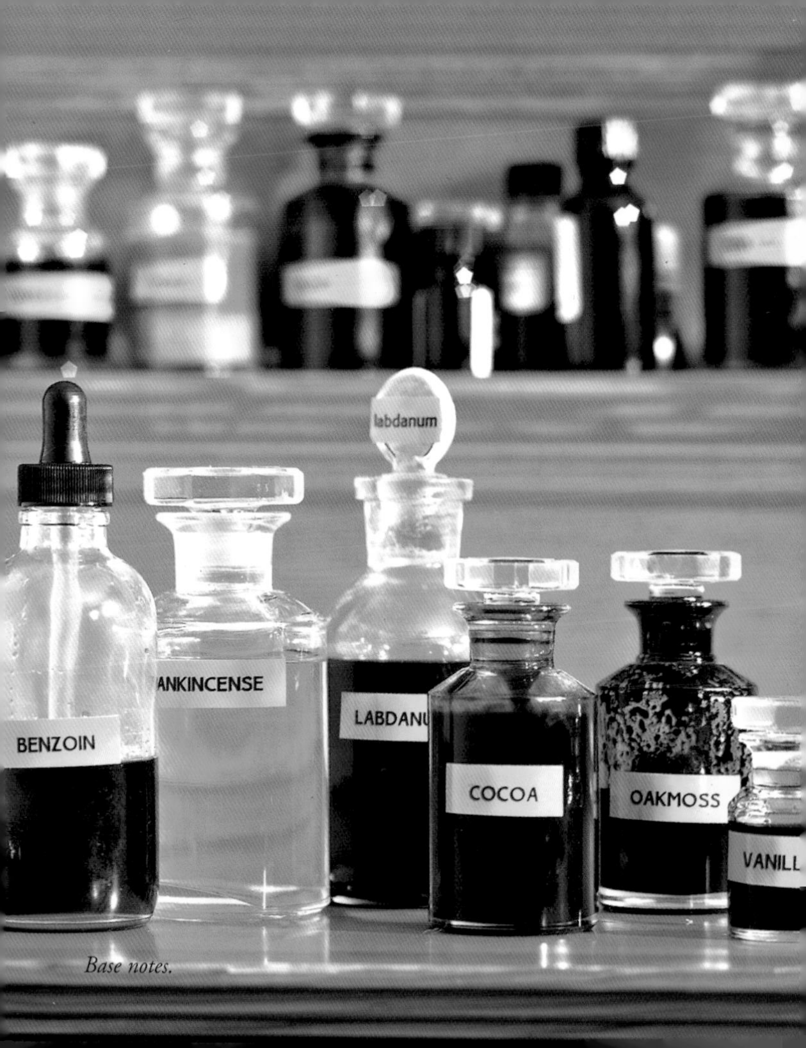

labdanum

BENZOIN

ANKINCENSE

LABDANUM

COCOA

OAKMOSS

VANILL

Base notes.

smelling slightly different. Usually essential oils smell sharper and lighter, absolutes are warmer and more voluptuous, and concretes are heavier and softer.

Top Notes (or Head Notes)

Here is a list of good top notes to start with; all of these are essential oils.

Bitter Orange

The bitter orange tree supplies the perfumer with an encyclopedia of scents—neroli and orange flower absolute from the blossoms, petitgrain oil from the leaves and twigs, and bitter orange essential oil from the peel of the fruit. The fresh, dry aroma has a rich and lasting sweet undertone. Though sharing similarities with other citruses, bitter orange has a different type of freshness, with a light floral undertone. It

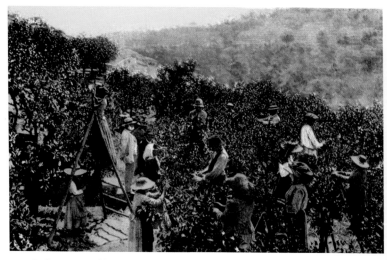

Picking orange blossoms.

is elegant and blends well with almost any other note; its aroma is positive and joyful, and just about everyone likes it. Store bitter orange essential oil in the refrigerator and replace every four months as it deteriorates.

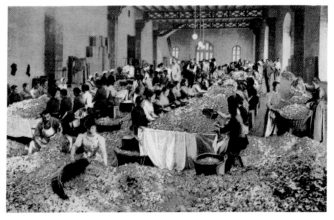

Sorting rose petals.

Bois de Rose

Bois de rose, or rosewood, distilled from the chipped wood of the *Aniba rosaeodora,* has a refreshing sweet, woody, spicy, somewhat rosy odor. Since there are almost no floral top notes, bois de rose is useful for creating a floral top note at the beginning of a perfume. It makes a good all-purpose top note that is uplifting, enlivening, and has an overall balancing effect.

Ginger

Ginger is considered by some to be the most ancient of all spices. Most ginger oil is distilled from dried roots, but the best essential oil is extracted from fresh ones. This pale-yellow to light-amber oil has sweet and heavy undertones that lend warmth and spiciness to a blend. The oil's initial fragrance resembles coriander mixed with lemon and orange, but it soon evolves to the warm, spicy scent of the root. Finally, ginger's dryout has slightly citrus undertones with fresh and woody notes. Ginger oil blends well with almost any other essence—the spices, woods, citruses, and florals. As an aphrodisiac, it is stimulating and warming.

Lime

The lime is a thorny, bushy evergreen tree with handsome dark green leaves so fragrant that they have been used to perfume the water in finger bowls. The rind of the fruit is cold-pressed to yield a greenish liquid that captures the rind's characteristically fresh, rich, sweet odor. Used moderately, it is mellow and "perfumey" and a good choice to finish off blends that are too sweet or too floral. Lime's aroma is refreshing and uplifting. Store lime essential oil in the refrigerator and replace every four months as it deteriorates.

Pink Grapefruit

My favorite grapefruit oil is cold-pressed from the peel of pink grapefruit. It is yellowish-orange in color, with a fresh, citrusy, rather sweet odor—sweeter, lighter, and more complicated than that of white grapefruit. Grapefruit is uplifting and reviving and blends well with basil, cedarwood, lavender, and ylang ylang. Store grapefruit essential oil in the refrigerator and replace every four months as it deteriorates.

Virginia Cedarwood

Virginia cedarwood is the wood used in lead pencils, and the oil is distilled from sawdust produced by pencil factories. Its scent starts out mild and pleasant, almost sweet and somewhat balsamic, like the wood itself, then becomes drier and woodier, less balsamic, as it moves toward the dryout note. Virginia cedarwood marries well with a variety of citruses and its aroma is elevating and strengthening.

Middle Notes (or Heart Notes)

These middle notes include concretes, absolutes, and essential oils.

Clary Sage Essential Oil

The green parts of the sage plant, especially the flowering tops, contain an essential oil with a delightful, somewhat wine-like odor. Clary sage starts out with a sweet, ambery, herbaceous note that progresses to a warm, balsamic dryout note. It imparts a mellowness, sweetness, and persistence to almost any perfume blend and is known for its calming, revitalizing, and balancing properties.

Jasmine Concrete

Jasmine is probably the most important perfume material. Its blossoms exhale a perfume so peculiar as

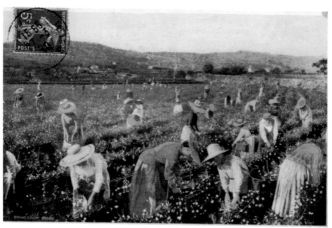

Harvesting jasmine.

to be incomparable. Synthetics do not even come close to approximating it. As with many flowers, jasmine blossoms continue to emit scent after they have been detached from the plant, and its character continues to develop until the blossoms fade and deteriorate. It takes a little more than two thousand pounds of flowers to produce a little less than two pounds of jasmine concrete. Rich and warm, heavy and fruity, intensely floral, it is almost narcotic in its ability to seize the senses and the imagination. Its almost cloying sweetness gives way to a drier note as it evolves, and it retains its warmth and depth all the way down to the dryout. There is almost no other essence with which jasmine does not beautifully blend, and no perfume that is not improved by its presence.

Jasmine concrete is a solid, reddish-orange wax whose sweet, mellow tone lends particular smoothness to any blend. Powerful as it is, jasmine refreshes rather than oppresses, possessing both antidepressant and aphrodisiacal properties.

Lavender Absolute

Lavender absolute, from the flowers and stalks of the lavender plant, is a beautiful dark green liquid with a pronounced herbaceous odor that dries down to a woody, spicy pungency like that of the flowering herb itself. The absolute is a much more interesting substance than the ubiquitous lavender oil, which, by comparison, seems thin and astringent. The absolute is particularly useful when you want a full-bodied lavender odor in the middle of a perfume, perhaps to lend an herbal note to a flowery middle accord. As a bonus, it lends a lovely hue to the finished perfume.

The aroma of lavender is restorative; it dispels anxiety and helps relieve stress and tension.

Nutmeg Absolute

Nutmeg absolute is deep orange, with a rounded sweet, warm, spicy aroma. Nutmeg's dryout is some-what woody but remains warm and sweet, without any sharpness. It is useful in spicy perfumes or to bring a sweet, warm note to any blend. Nutmeg is known to invigorate and stimulate the mind.

Rose Absolute

Roses and their essences possess infinite variation. It has even been noted that the roses on a given bush smell different at different times of day, and the intensity of

Rose is thought to drive away melancholy and lift and open the heart.

the scent increases before a storm. Therefore, the blossoms are gathered before they open, a little before sunrise. Were they gathered later in the day, in full flower, the perfume would be stronger but not as sweet.

Rose absolute, like jasmine, mixes well with any other oil. It forgives all indiscretions and brings out the best in the other notes with its full-bodied, unthreatening beauty. If you have made a mistake in your blending, sometimes adding a bit more rose will remedy the problem. My favorite of all the rose absolutes is Moroccan rose, with its complex but soft and sweet scent.

Needless to say, rose is an aphrodisiac. It is also thought to drive away melancholy and lift and open the heart.

Ylang Ylang Concrete

Ylang ylang, "flower of flowers," has been dubbed a poor man's jasmine. To me it is the definition of a good buy, inexpensive and beautiful. Ylang ylang concrete is so multilayered it is perfume on its own—a creamy, sweet note that is suave, soft, and persistent. Ylang ylang is one of the most important raw materials for perfume. Dosed with discretion, it produces remarkable effects, imparting floral top notes as well as middle notes. It blends well with jasmine and rose, bergamot and vanilla.

Ylang ylang is an aphrodisiac that relieves tension and imparts joy.

Base Notes

These base notes are derived from resins, absolutes, and essential oils.

Benzoin Resin

Benzoin is a secretion of the tree *Styrax tonkinense*. The trees do not produce the secretion naturally, however. A wound is inflicted in the bark deep enough to result in the formation of ducts through which the resinous secretion is produced. When it is sufficiently hard and dry, the material is collected in the form of small lumps or tears. Benzoin has a soft, sweet, warm body note that evolves into a balsamic powdery finish and blends with almost anything. It is a good fixative for oriental scents and, to a lesser extent, florals. It is an inexpensive one, as well, and can be used economically to extend a vanilla note.

People tend to find benzoin calming, seductive, sensual, and rejuvenating.

Cocoa Absolute

Cocoa absolute *(Theobroma cacao)* is a dark brown thick absolute extracted from cocoa beans. Some cocoa absolutes are sweeter, some richer, some more bitter, like the varieties of dark chocolate. Cocoa absolute blends well with the obvious chocolate partners—mint, orange, vanilla—as well as ylang

ylang, saffron, and jasmine. The scent of chocolate has always been thought of as an aphrodisiac.

Frankincense Essential Oil

Frankincense is found in the bark of various small trees of the *Boswellia* genus. In ancient times it was, without a doubt, the most important perfume substance. Frankincense has a soft, incense-like odor. It remains an important and elegant fixative in spicy, exotic, and flowery perfumes, and it works well with citruses also. Frankincense is a diffusive, lighter base note that can blend with milder notes without dominating them. It has an elevating and soothing effect on the mind.

Labdanum Absolute

Labdanum is the resinous exudation of rockrose *(Cistus ladaniferus)*, a small shrub that grows wild around the Mediterranean. Long ago, the oleoresin was collected by shepherds, who combed it from the fleece of sheep that had been browsing among cistus bushes. These days, the twigs and leaves of the plant are boiled in water to yield the aromatic gum. Labdanum has a pronounced sweet, herbaceous, balsamic odor, with a rich amber undertone found in few other essences. Labdanum, the principle amber aroma, is comforting and centering.

Oakmoss Absolute

True oakmoss *(mousse de chêne)* is the soft, treacly, greenish-black lichen *Evernia prunastri,* which grows primarily on oak trees. In its natural state it has no discernible fragrance, but after it has dried and rested for a while, it develops a scent reminiscent of seashore, bark, wood, and foliage. In sparing doses, it lends the scent of a wet forest to the dryout note of a perfume, giving the whole a naturalness and a rich, earthy undertone. It is also a great fixative. Oakmoss requires restraint on the part of the perfumer; too much can ruin a creation.

Deep and profound, the aroma of oakmoss is grounding.

Vanilla Absolute

The vanilla plant is an orchid, a vine that climbs along tree trunks. Its seedpod exhales one of the finest odors in the vegetable kingdom. The culture and preparation of vanilla involves a kind of alchemy, however. The seedpod has no fragrance when it is gathered, but develops its characteristic odor as it ferments during the curing process, under the sorcery of sun and air. The lower end of the pod begins to turn yellow and it releases a penetrating scent of bitter almonds. By degrees the color darkens, the flesh softens, and the true odor of vanilla begins to develop as the natural fermentation gradually progresses up the pod. The scent of vanilla is universally beloved and there is no essence that it does not combine with beautifully. Vanilla can also sometimes be used as an accessory note to enliven bitter blends.

Most people find the smell of vanilla to be an aphrodisiac—it is comforting and reassuring.

$\mathcal{E}$QUIPMENT $\mathscr{C}$ SUPPLIES

*T*HE EQUIPMENT YOU WILL NEED to begin making perfume is simple and readily available, as well as easy to use. Many of these items you will already have in your kitchen; for the others I have given sources at the end of the book.

Measuring Equipment

Droppers. They are used for measuring essences and other ingredients and can be bought a drugstore or by the dozen at chemical supply houses. I prefer these to the orifice-reducer dropper caps that come

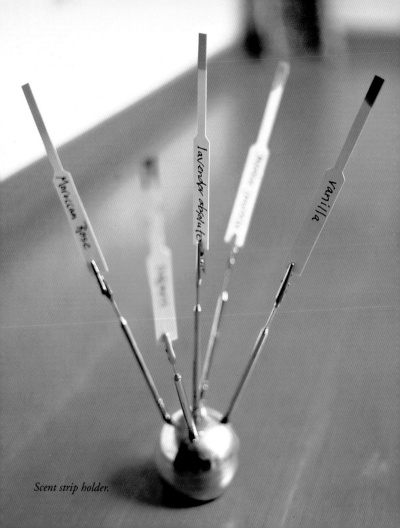

Scent strip holder.

with many essences; they give you greater control and less risk of error. With essences of high odor intensity, one drop too many can ruin everything. I always use glass droppers, never plastic pipettes.

1 small scoop. A bamboo scoop (sold in China Towns as a scoop to clear ears) or crochet hook is a useful way to measure solid concretes. A scoop the size of a very small pea ● is equal to one drop. Be sure to clean your scoop in alcohol after each use.

10-ml beaker. This is used for blending your perfume ingredients. The "low form" (chubby) beakers give you the ability to vigorously mash concrete material into your blend and to smell your creation as it evolves.

Measuring spoons. They are used for larger quantities of ingredients. An ordinary plastic or metal set used for cooking is fine.

Most of the beakers for measuring fragrance ingredients are calibrated in metric measurements. In case you do not have this kind of beaker, I have translated the metric so you can use measuring spoons instead.

$$ml = milliliters$$
$$.6\ ml = \tfrac{1}{8}\ teaspoon$$
$$1.25\ ml = \tfrac{1}{4}\ teaspoon$$
$$2.5\ ml = \tfrac{1}{2}\ teaspoon$$
$$3.75\ ml = \tfrac{3}{4}\ teaspoon$$
$$5\ ml = 1\ teaspoon$$
$$15\ ml = 1\ tablespoon$$

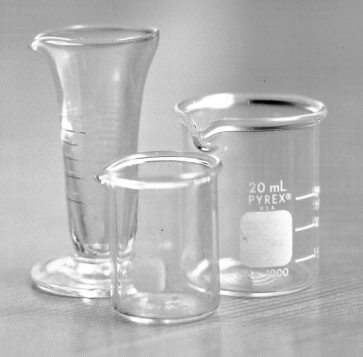

Small beakers.

Tools

Fragrance testing strips. These are essential tools for exploring the world of odors. I particularly like the paddle-shaped strips because they give you ample room for labeling. Write the name of the material you are sampling on the thicker end and dip the other end a half inch into the material itself, then smell.

Bamboo skewers. These are used for stirring. The skewers need to be cut down so they don't topple out of the beakers. Small salt spoons are perfect for mixing solid perfumes.

Small adhesive labels for your bottles. I like to use circular labels—white ones for experiments and colored ones for my bottles of essences. (I use yellow for top notes, orange for middle notes, and green for base notes.) Be sure to label both the cap and bottom of each bottle in case one of the labels falls off or you have many caps off at one time.

Grater. A simple grater is used for grating beeswax. The trapezoidal kind you use for cheese is fine. I use the medium-sized holes and grate a cup at a time. Store the grated beeswax in a resealable plastic bag.

Nonmetal pan. This is used for melting wax. Ceramic or glass is best, the smaller the better. A small ramekin or soufflé dish is suitable. Chemical supply houses sell extremely tiny heat-proof ceramic pans called "casseroles" that, while not essential, are perfect for the small batches of wax used in solid perfume.

Gas or electric burner. This is the heat source for melting the wax. If you really get into making solid perfume, it is extremely useful to get a small hot plate from a laboratory supply company. Choose a small, portable one with an easy-to-clean ceramic top.

Containers for solid perfumes. A container for solid perfume should be round, oval, or square, but not triangular because it is hard to get the perfume out of the corners. I prefer small compacts, not as large as the ones regularly found in department stores. Shallow containers are also preferable, because it is difficult to get the perfume out of a deeper basin. Small compacts and pillboxes are perfect, and they are easy to find at flea markets or online. A secure latch or lid is important. Old metal compacts work well, as do silver, enamel, or porcelain pillboxes. You can also use small jars or lip-balm containers.

Supplies

Beeswax. I prefer natural yellow beeswax, which I purchase in one-pound blocks—this is enough to last most home perfumers for many years. It lends a sweetish fragrance and a warm amber glow to solid perfumes, and the process of grating it, melting it, and smelling its delicate honeyed scent contributes to the meditative aspects of making perfume. Bleached beeswax is also available, but I do not recommend it—the texture is thin, the bleaching gives the wax a chemical smell, and the resulting perfume is pasty in texture and appearance.

Jojoba Oil. This is actually a wax, not a liquid oil, that closely resembles human sebum and is therefore

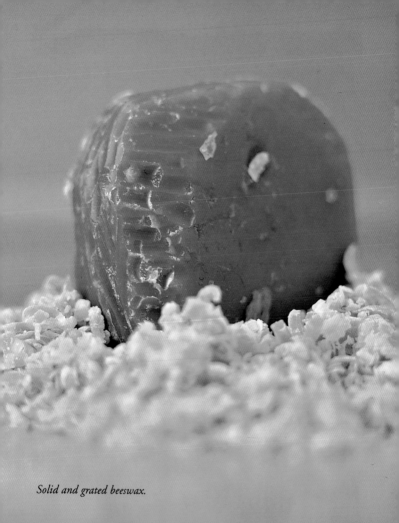

Solid and grated beeswax.

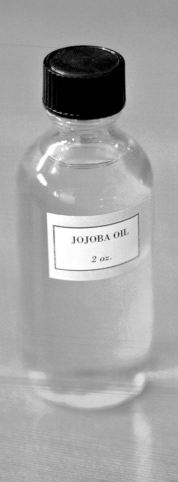

an excellent moisturizer. It comes from the seeds of a desert shrub and is a lovely golden color, with no fragrance of its own; it is also much less prone to rancidity and oxidation than other oils.

Rubbing Alcohol. This is used for cleaning droppers and is easily obtained in any drugstore.

Your Blend of Natural Essences. These will vary with the perfume you are making.

CREATING SOLID PERFUMES

SOLID PERFUME IS CREATED BY combining the right amounts of beeswax, jojoba oil, and essences over heat and then pouring the mixture into a container where it can set to the proper consistency. In this chapter you will learn the basics of making solid perfumes, as well as recipes specifically designed to enhance your sense of well-being.

Essentials of Solid Perfume

Creating solid perfumes is a great place to begin as a perfumer. Solid perfumes are very forgiving and with

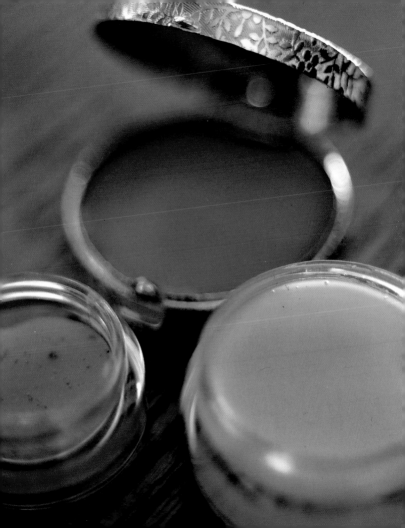

practice anyone can create a good one. A solid perfume can be very beautiful with just two or three essences. You can even create a solid perfume from only one essence. This simple solid can be layered over other perfumes or worn alone. Nothing could be simpler!

Note: You can create a single-note solid perfume from middle or base notes but not from top notes. The jojoba oil and beeswax hold down the top notes, so a solid perfume created from only top notes will not evolve properly and will disappear immediately from the skin.

The proper ratio of beeswax to jojoba oil is what creates the texture of a good solid perfume; the texture should be similar to that of a good lipstick—creamy, but firm enough to offer some resistance, yet not so hard that it takes any real force to get some to adhere. Apply solid perfume by running the ball of your finger back and forth across the surface of the perfume. Do not use your fingertip to scoop it out, as this leaves an unsightly marred surface on the perfume.

Olfactory Fatigue

Whenever you work with natural perfume materials, beware of olfactory fatigue, which can set in after you smell too many scents in a row. When essences begin to smell weak, I know it is time to refresh the olfactory palate. The easiest way to do this is to inhale three times deeply through a piece of wool—a scarf or shawl works well—which revitalizes your sense of smell.

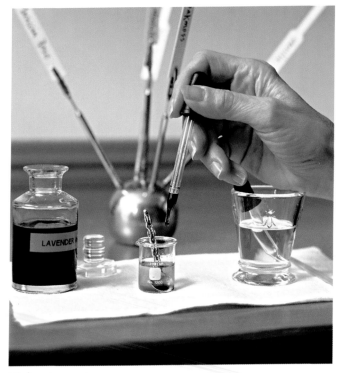

Work environment.

Setting Up Your Work Environment

Fold a paper towel in half. Put the beaker or bowl you are going to use for mixing on the left side. On the right, place a shot glass filled with rubbing alcohol or perfume alcohol and droppers. Add the correct amount of jojoba to the receptacle on the left. Drop by drop, add the essences of the formula to the

---

Natural fragrance always blossoms on the body and should be smelled on your skin.

---

jojoba oil, always adding base notes first, then middle notes, and finally top notes. If you add the base notes last you will not be able to smell the top notes clearly or understand their effect on a blend.

Smell the perfume after each addition. Do this by putting a drop on your hand; natural fragrance always blossoms on the body and should be smelled on your skin. By smelling after each addition, you will be able to experience the aromatic changes each essence brings to the blend.

Have all your materials out and available when you are "cooking" a solid perfume, and do not allow any distractions or interruptions or you may overheat the blend.

Working with Solid Materials

Solid or semisolid essences like labdanum, oakmoss, and jasmine require a scoop for measuring them out. I use a bamboo scoop, but a small crochet hook will work well too. Simply scoop out a piece of the material about the size of a very small pea ● and consider that one drop.

Creating Solid Perfumes

Use the following recipes to create solid perfumes especially for you. Experiment with the different essences and recipes to see what you like best. The process of making the perfume, as well as wearing it, can do a great deal toward enhancing your sense of well-being.

❧ BASIC SOLID PERFUME RECIPE

5 ml jojoba oil

20 drops of essence

½ *heaping* tsp. grated beeswax

Small nonmetal pan for melting wax

Lip-balm jar or compact for finished perfume

Pour 5 ml jojoba oil into a beaker or small bowl or cup. Add twenty drops of your perfume formula into the jojoba oil. Melt the ½ heaping teaspoon of beeswax in a nonmetal pan or dish over heat. Remove from heat and stir in the perfume blend. Return to heat for around 5 seconds and stir to combine. (Do not overheat the wax or the essences.) Immediately pour the mixture into a container and let it set, undisturbed, for 15 minutes.

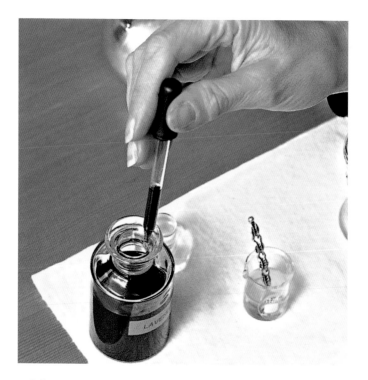

Fill dropper with absolute.

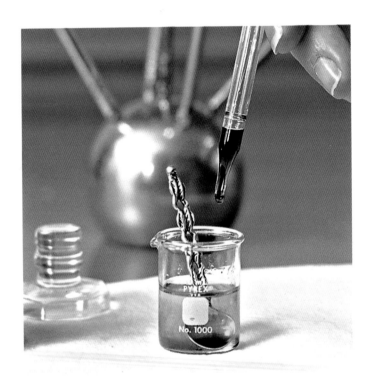

Drop absolute into jojoba oil.

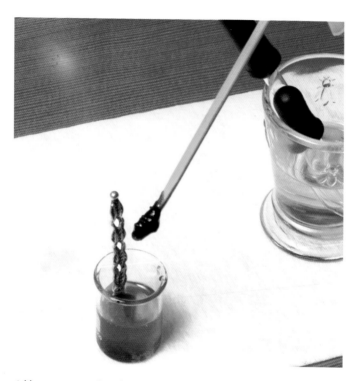

Add concrete to jojoba oil.

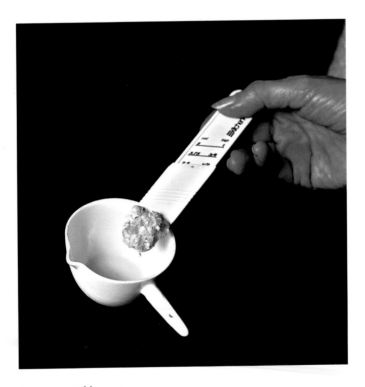

Measure grated beeswax.

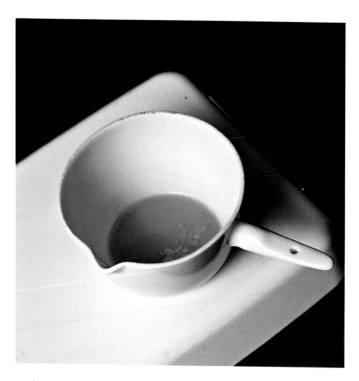

Melt wax.

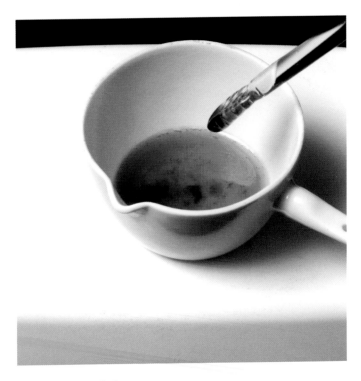

Stir essence into melted wax.

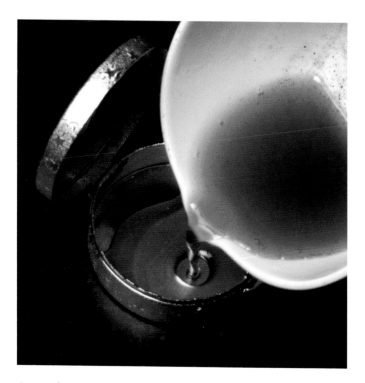

Pour perfume mixture into compact.

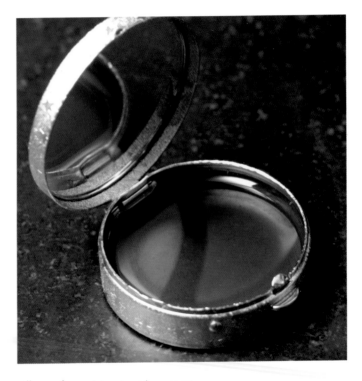

Allow perfume mixture to set in compact.

Simple Recipes for Well-Being

You can create a simple one-note solid perfume with any of the following essences, all of which are known to affect the emotions:

For *tranquility* try one of the following:
- 20 drops clary sage
- 20 drops lavender absolute
- 20 drops benzoin
- 20 drops frankincense
- 10 drops oakmoss

For *joy* try one of the following:
- 20 drops ylang ylang concrete
- 20 drops rose absolute

For sensuality try one of the following:

- 20 drops jasmine absolute
- 20 drops vanilla absolute
- 20 drops labdanum
- 20 drops cocoa absolute

More Complex Recipes for Well-Being

You can create more complex solid perfumes with the following recipes:

For a sense of uplifting refreshment, combine the following essences:

- 4 drops nutmeg absolute, 10 drops Virginia cedarwood, 6 drops lime
- 5 drops bitter orange, 10 drops bois de rose, 5 drops lavender absolute

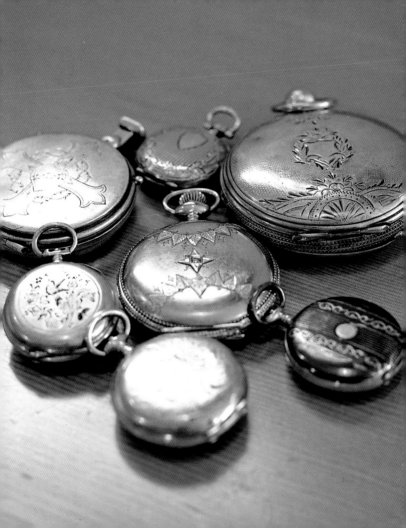

For a sense of tranquility, combine the following essences:

- 7 drops clary sage, 13 drops benzoin
- 6 drops lavender absolute, 12 drops frankincense, 2 drops oakmoss

For a sense of joy, combine the following essences:

- 15 drops grapefruit, 5 drops ylang ylang
- 8 drops bois de rose, 8 drops bitter orange, 4 drops jasmine

For a sense of sensuality, combine the following essences:

- 7 drops jasmine, 8 drops labdanum, 5 drops cocoa
- 7 drops ginger, 10 drops vanilla, 3 drops cocoa absolute

Enjoy the recipes on the previous pages or experiment with your own combinations. The pleasure of making your own solid perfumes can be addictive, and the joy of wearing them is a simple and fulfilling way to add a measure of well-being to your life.

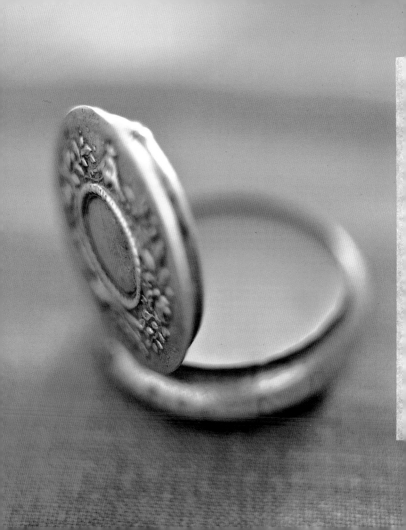

RESOURCES

Contact Aftelier Perfumes for natural perfumes (both solid and liquid), *The Natural Perfume Workbook and Wheel,* and essential oils, absolutes, and concretes. Aftelier also offers perfume essence and equipment kits that include everything you need to make solid perfumes.

Aftelier Perfumes
510.841.2111
www.aftelier.com

Essential Oils, Absolutes, and Concretes
The Essential Oil University
812.945.5000
www.essentialoils.org

Liberty Natural Products
800.289.8427
www.libertynatural.com

Millefiori
www.mille-fiori.net

John Steele/Lifetree Aromatix
818.986.0594

Sunrose Aromatics
718.794.0391
www.sunrosearomatics.com

White Lotus Aromatics
FAX: 510.528.9441
www.whitelotusaromatics.com

Lab Equipment
VWR catalogue
800.932.5000
www.vwr.com

Scent Strips and Jojoba Oil
Liberty Natural Products
800.289.8427
www.libertynatural.com

Organic Beeswax
Glory Bee Foods
800.456.7923
www.GlotyBeeFoods.com

*Small Compacts and Lockets
for Solid Perfume*
Eli Metal Products Company
800.552.4554